The Scientific Approach to Exercise for Fat Loss

How to Get In Shape and Shed Unwanted Fat

A Review of Healthy and Scientifically Proven Techniques

PAUL ORRIDGE BSc

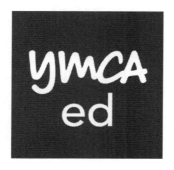

Discover more books and ebooks of interest to you and find out about the range of work we do at the forefront of health, fitness and wellbeing.

www.centralymcaguides.com

Published by Central YMCA Trading Ltd (trading as YMCAed).
Registered Company No. 3667206.

Central YMCA is the world's founding YMCA. Established in 1844 in Central London, it was the first YMCA to open its doors and, in so doing, launched a movement that has now grown to become the world's biggest youth organisation. Today, Central YMCA is the UK's leading health, fitness and wellbeing charity, committed to helping people from all walks of life – and particularly the young and those with a specific need – to live happier, healthier and more fulfilled lives.

Copyright © Central YMCA Trading Ltd 2013
All rights reserved.

ISBN: 1481905147
ISBN-13: 978-1481905145

All rights reserved. No part of this publication may be reproduced, stored in a retrieval system, or transmitted, in any form or by any means, without the prior permission of the publisher. This book is presented solely for educational and entertainment purposes. The author and publisher are not offering it as legal, medical, or other professional services advice. While best efforts have been used in preparing this book, the author and publisher make no representations or warranties of any kind and assume no liabilities of any kind with respect to the accuracy or completeness of the contents and specifically disclaim any implied warranties of merchantability or fitness of use for a particular purpose. Neither the publisher nor the individual author(s) shall be liable for any physical, psychological, emotional, financial, or commercial damages, including, but not limited to, special, incidental, consequential or other damages, resulting from the information or programs contained herein. Every person is different and the information, advice and programs contained herein may not be suitable for your situation. Exercise is not without its risks and, as such, we would strongly advise that you consult with your healthcare professional before beginning any programme of exercise, especially if you have, or suspect you may have, any injuries or illnesses, are currently pregnant or have recently given birth. The advice, information and guidance given in Central YMCA Guides is in no way intended as a substitute for medical consultation. As with any form of exercise, you should stop immediately if you feel faint, dizzy or have physical discomfort or pain or any other contra indication, and consult a physician.

CONTENTS

About The Author

	Introduction	1
1	The Size Of The Problem	3
2	The Physiology Of Fat	7
3	Nature Versus Nurture: Why We Get Fatter	13
4	Planning Your Fat Loss Programme	19
5	Creating Your Fat Burning Programme	27
6	In Conclusion	41
7	References and Further Information	43
	The Central YMCA Guides Series	51

ABOUT THE AUTHOR

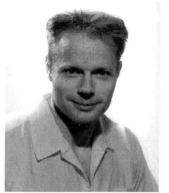

Paul Orridge BSc(Hons) has a first class honours degree in exercise and health and over 20 years' experience within the fitness industry. In this time he has performed a variety of roles including personal training, lecturing and writing. As personal trainer, Paul has conducted several thousand training sessions, and has taught over two thousand exercise professionals. He has developed and presented a variety of fitness related courses for a number of industry providers.

Paul's work is based on his practical experience gained working with a diverse range of people from very unfit, overweight individuals to highly conditioned elite athletes, and is underpinned by the latest research.

Paul keeps himself fit with a combination of running, kayaking and resistance training. Paul's other interests including reading and music. Before pursuing a career in the fitness industry, Paul worked as professional musician.

INTRODUCTION

Turn on the television or open any typical lifestyle magazine today and you are likely to be confronted by images of fit, lean looking people promoting a vast array of different products, from razors and shampoos to breakfast cereals and holiday homes. Similarly, the covers of popular fitness magazines are often plastered with images of rippling torsos and the promise of a quick and easy way of achieving the perfect body. Terms such as 'ripped' and 'shredded' are commonplace, as are diet and exercise plans that promise to get you into your bikini in a fortnight. Based on these examples you could be forgiven for thinking that we are all generally lean and active and just in need of a little help to achieve the 'six-pack' or waistline of our dreams. The reality, however, is very different.

In this book we will take a scientific look at the myths and misunderstandings around body fat, healthy lifestyles and exercise, separating fact from fiction and providing you with a proven way to achieve healthy body fat levels safely and effectively.

Based on the findings of the latest scientific research and guidelines from the most highly regarded health organisations, we'll show you how to develop an exercise programme to help you achieve a healthy level of body fat in the safest and most effective way.

Simple, effective and scientifically proven. Forget the crash diets and exercise fads, here's what you really need to know.

Central YMCA Health and Fitness Guides

1

THE SIZE OF THE PROBLEM

Have you found yourself requiring fewer holes in your belts of late? Or have the buttons on your shirt become harder to do up in recent months? Perhaps you've put it down to a 'contented' lifestyle, or the dreaded middle-age spread. Whatever the reasons, you're certainly not alone in experiencing an increase in the level of your body fat.

Worldwide obesity rates have more than doubled since 1980. Indeed, the World Health Organization (WHO, 2012) has described the problem of obesity as an 'epidemic' and one of the fastest growing health problems today.

In 2008, more than 1.4 billion adults were classified as overweight. Of these, over 200 million men and nearly 300 million women were obese. Furthermore, it is predicted that by the year 2015, 2.15 billion adults will be overweight and 700 million will be obese (WHO, 2008). To put this rising trend in obesity into perspective, the average man was 7.7kg (17lb) heavier in the year 2000 than he was in 1986. Women, meanwhile, had an average weight gain of 5.4 kg (12lb) (Scarborough et al., 2010).

Excessively high levels of body fat not only affect the way a person looks but can also have a profound impact on their health, as they greatly increase the chances of developing a considerable number of health problems. These can include cardiovascular disease, pulmonary disease, type 2 diabetes, osteoarthritis, certain cancers (breast, uterus and colon) and mental health conditions (ACSM, 2006). At least 2.8 million adults die each year as a result of being overweight or obese (WHO, 2012).

The link between high levels of body fat and poor health is not a recent discovery; it has been acknowledged for centuries. Indeed, the historians amongst you may be interested to know that Hippocrates (460 -377 BC), the 'Father of Medicine', stated that obesity is a health risk and considered it a cause of disease that led to death (McArdle et al., 2010).

The fundamental cause of this 'epidemic' is generally acknowledged as an energy imbalance between the amount of calories consumed and the amount expended (WHO, 2012). Unlike many other epidemics, the 'cure' for the obesity epidemic is well known. If you ask the average person what you need to do to reduce fat levels they will probably say something about reducing the amount we eat, making 'healthier' food choices and increasing the amount of physical activity we do.

So if the cause and the cure are known, why are body fat levels still rising?

Although reducing body fat seems straightforward, many people have incorporated patterns of overeating, poor food choices and physical inactivity into their lifestyle. In an effort to reduce body fat levels quickly, people often turn to fad diets and inappropriate exercise regimens which are often ineffective and difficult to maintain, resulting in a return to old habits and an increase in body fat.

There is evidence to suggest that only 50% of people trying to reduce their levels of body fat use the recommended method of restricting calorie intake and increasing physical activity levels (Heyward, 2006). Of those people who do engage in physical activity to reduce their body fat levels, only 20% meet the guidelines for physical activity (30 minutes of activity on most days of the week, or preferably daily), which is about half the amount needed (Heyward, 2006).

Ironically, the rise in obesity levels has been accompanied by a dramatic rise in eating disorders such as anorexia and bulimia. At least 1.1 million people in the UK and up to 24 million people in the United States are affected by some form of eating disorder (Disordered Eating, 2011).

Research has shown that eating disorders are caused by a complex interplay between genetics, family history and the cultural environment. The media, however, commonly portray images of attractiveness that can influence people's perceptions of acceptable body image. The images of slim, often unhealthy, lean models in the media are a stark contrast to the body size, shape and composition of the people to whom the images are aimed; people who are becoming increasingly fatter (BMA, 2000). Consequently, we have a situation in which we are getting fatter but view individuals with often unrealistic or unhealthily low levels of body fat as role models.

The key to successfully achieving and maintaining healthy levels of body fat is the adoption of a healthy lifestyle: eating the appropriate types and amounts of food and doing the right types and amounts of physical activity (Heyward, 2006).

In the next chapter, we will look at how our body fat stores increase.

2

THE PHYSIOLOGY OF FAT

The subject of fat loss goes hand in hand with an array of misconceptions. For example, a common misunderstanding is that fat *per se* is bad. Wrong. We all need to eat certain types of fat in the appropriate amounts and maintain a certain level of body fat for general good health. Body fat is also a vital source of energy, even for lean people. The body fat stores of a person with 12% body fat would typically exceed 70,000kcals, enough energy to run 700 miles (Wilmore et al., 2008; McArdle et al., 2010). In order to develop a safe and effective fat loss programme, we therefore need to have some understanding of the role of body fat in our health and the physiological processes that occur when we increase and decrease our levels of body fat.

ENERGY AND FAT

To understand how we gain and lose body fat we need to understand the concept of energy.

All of our energy originates from the sun in the form of light. Plants then convert light energy into stored chemical energy, which we obtain by eating the plants, or by eating the animals that eat the plants. This energy is stored in our food as carbohydrate, protein and fat, which we break down to provide us with energy (Wilmore et al., 2008).

This food-derived energy is then used for various functions in our bodies, such as growth and repair of tissues, the transportation of substances and, of course, to fuel skeletal muscle activity to produce movement.

Muscle activity can place a huge stress on the body's ability to produce energy. The rate at which we expend energy when we're exercising at full capacity, such as when we're sprinting for even a few seconds, can be much greater than that which we expel when we're resting (Wilmore and Costill, 2004).

Energy that our bodies don't use tends to get stored as fat.

CALORIES

Whether you count them or watch them, one term that always tends to occur in any discussion on fat loss is *calorie*. But what is a calorie? Think of it this way. All energy ultimately becomes heat and one calorie is simply the heat energy needed to increase the temperature of 1 gram of water by 1° C, specifically from 14.5 to 15.5° C. To describe the energy content of food and the energy expenditure of the body we use the term kilocalories (kcal); one kcal is 1000 calories. This equals the amount of heat energy needed to raise 1 kilogram of water by 1° C, from 14.5 to 15.5° C (McArdle et al., 2010).

If you look on food labels you will see that different foods contain different amounts of potential energy (Wilmore et al., 2008). For example, half a cup of peanut butter has the energy value of 759kcal, which is the equivalent heat energy to increase the temperature of 759 litres of water by one degree (McArdle et al., 2010).

One gram of fat, meanwhile, provides approximately 9 kcal. Protein and carbohydrate have an energy content of approximately 4kcal/g, with alcohol providing 7kcal/g (Wilmore et al., 2008).
All this science essentially means that although high-fat foods have the potential to provide us with greater amounts of energy, which, if not used, can ultimately become body fat, energy from any food source has the potential of becoming body fat.

HOW DO OUR BODY FAT LEVELS INCREASE AND DECREASE?

Our bodies store fat in specialised cells known as adipocytes or fat cells. Typically, when we gain moderate amounts of weight, due to consuming more energy than we use, existing fat cells tend to fill up with more fat and become enlarged in a process called fat cell hypertrophy (Heyward, 2006).
In cases of severe obesity, in which already obese people gain even greater

amounts of body fat, the fat cells reach a limit beyond which they cannot increase in size. At this point, the *number* of fat cells can increase in a process called fat cell hyperplasia (McArdle et al., 2010).

The level of obesity required to result in an increase in the number of adipocytes is believed to be around 60% body fat or about 170% of normal weight (McArdle et al., 1996).

When we reduce our body fat stores, the individual fat cells shrink but there is no decrease in their number (McArdle et al., 2010).

WHERE IS BODY FAT STORED?

When we think of where are body fat is stored we tend think of the areas that are easily visible, such as the abdominal area or the thighs. However, it is a little more complex than that. Body fat is stored in two sites referred to as essential fat and storage fat.

Essential fat consists of the fat stored in the marrow of our bones and our organs, such as the heart, liver, spleen, kidneys, the muscles and the central nervous system. As the name suggests, this fat is essential for maintaining a healthy body. Women have sex-specific essential fat in their breasts, pelvis, thigh and buttock regions, which is important for hormonal functions and child bearing.

Storage fat consists of the fat that protects the organs within the chest and abdomen from trauma, and the fat under the surface of the skin, which tends to be the fat that people are most concerned with (McArdle et al., 2010).

Men and women have similar proportions of storage fat (12% of body mass in men and 15% in women), but the percentage of essential fat in women, which includes the sex-specific fat, is typically four times greater than in men (McArdle et al., 2010). Consequently, women need a greater amount of body fat for good health than men. This has to be kept in mind when setting your fat loss goal.

ARE YOU AN APPLE OR A PEAR?

Where we carry our body fat, regardless of how much total body fat we have, is generally acknowledged as an important predictor of the health risks associated with obesity.

If you are an apple shape, where your body fat is mainly deposited on your abdomen, you have a greater risk of developing a number of different health problems, such as hypertension, type 2 diabetes and coronary heart disease compared to those who are a pear shape, in which the fat is deposited on the hips and thighs (Heyward, 2006; Mayo Clinic, 2011). This is because abdominal fat is not just limited to the layer located just below the skin (subcutaneous fat). It also includes visceral fat, which lies deep inside your abdomen, surrounding your internal organs. An excessive amount of visceral fat produces hormones and other substances that can raise blood pressure, negatively alter cholesterol levels and impair the body's ability to use insulin (Mayo Clinic, 2011).

When gaining body fat men tend to be more apple shaped, which is referred to as android obesity. Women, on the other hand, tend to be more pear shaped, referred to as gynoid obesity. However, some men have gynoid obesity and some women have android obesity (Heyward, 2006). Women tend to gain more fat on their abdomen after the menopause, when fat tends to shift from the arms, legs and hips to this area (Mayo, 2011).

WHY DO WE PUT FAT ON IN DIFFERENT PLACES?

You may be a person who tends to gain fat on their abdominal area, or perhaps it goes on your thighs or bottom. The substance responsible for these differences between individuals in their fat deposits is lipoprotein lipase (LPL). This facilitates fat uptake and storage by the fat cells. The differences in fat distribution seen between men and women are also related to the larger amount of LPL possessed by women. The fat cells of the hip, thigh and breast region produce considerable amounts in women; whereas in males, the abdominal fat cells are active with this fat-storing substance (McArdle et al., 1996). Consequently, when men gain body fat it tends to go on their abdomens, while women tend to gain it on the hips, thighs and breasts.

When obese people reduce their body fat, the level of LPL in their fat cells increases. The fatter a person is before fat loss, the greater the amount of LPL produced when fat is lost. This makes it easier for formerly obese people to regain body fat. Unfortunately, it seems the fatter a person is initially, the more vigorously their body tries to regain the lost fat (McArdle et al., 2010).

CAN EXERCISE 'SPOT REDUCE' BODY FAT?

It may seem logical that if we carry fat in a certain area of the body then by exercising that part we could reduce the fat in that area. For example, a common belief is that performing abdominal exercises will specifically reduce the level of fat on the abdomen. However, the results of numerous studies (Carns et al., 1960; Norland and Kearney, 1978; Roby, 1962; Achade et al., 1962; Katch et al., 1984; Despres et al., 1985 cited in Heyward, 2006) have shown that spot reduction exercises are no more effective than general aerobic exercise for reducing body fat levels.

In fact, a 20-week cycling programme reduced abdominal fat stores to a greater degree than those of the legs (Despres et al., 1985 cited in Heyward, 1991). If spot reduction worked, one would expect the fat stores of the legs to be more affected by cycling than those of the abdomen. The idea of spot reduction is very attractive for both cosmetic and health reasons, but the research shows it doesn't work (McArdle et al., 2010).

It is clear that we need a certain amount of body fat, as it plays a number of important roles in our bodies, including being a source of energy, protecting vital organs and insulating us against the cold. However, having too much body fat or too little, or carrying it the wrong place can be detrimental to our health.

In the next chapter, we will look at the theories regarding why our body fat levels increase and why some people are more prone than others to gaining body fat.

3

NATURE VERSUS NURTURE: WHY WE GET FATTER

How often have you overheard people discussing body fat and professing, 'I can eat whatever I want and I don't put on an ounce' or, on the other hand, 'I only have to walk past a cake shop and I put on a pound'?

Clearly some people do struggle more than others to achieve and maintain healthy levels of body fat. Hormone problems or genetics are often cited as the cause of a person's excess fat, but how big an influence are these factors, can they explain the dramatic rise in obesity levels in the last 30 years and is there any such thing as being big boned?

WHAT ROLE DO HORMONES PLAY?

The short answer to this question is not a lot. Indeed, only around one case in every 1,000 of obesity is caused by a hormonal problem (Sharkey, 1990).

One example of how this rare incidence can occur is when the amount of energy our bodies use at rest, known as resting metabolic rate, is reduced by as much as 30-50% through underproduction of the hormone thyroxine from the thyroid gland (Heyward, 1991).

To put this in perspective, if a person normally burns 1,800kcal per day at rest, a reduction in thyroxine levels could reduce this to 900 to 1260 kcal per day. If their energy intake (food and drink) and physical activity levels remain unchanged, however, this is equivalent to consuming an extra 540 to

900 kcal per day or 3,780 to 6,300 kcal per week! This positive energy balance will therefore inevitably cause an increase in body fat (Heyward, 2006).

ARE OUR GENES MAKING OUR JEANS TIGHTER?

Hardly a week passes without the media reporting a new breakthrough in our understanding of the role genetics play in the development of many diseases, including obesity. For example, research has shown that people carrying one copy of a gene known as FTO have a 30% increased risk of being obese, compared to a person with no copies. A person carrying two copies of the gene, meanwhile, has a 70% increased risk of being obese than a similar person with no copies. And if you thought that the chances of carrying two copies are slim, think again. Approximately 16% of people of European descent carry two copies of this genetic variant and are on average 3kg heavier than those without (Church et al., 2010).

Our genes could predispose us to gaining body fat in a number of ways. Obesity-related genes may affect how we metabolise food or store fat. They could also affect our behaviour, making us inclined towards lifestyle choices that increase our risk of being obese. For example, people with variations in certain 'obesity genes' tend to eat more meals and snacks, consume more calories per day, and often choose the same types of high fat, sugary foods (Lifespan, 2012).

Other genes, meanwhile, may control appetite, making us less able to sense when we are full. Some may make us more responsive to the taste, smell or sight of food, or perhaps affect our sense of taste, giving us preferences for high fat foods, or putting us off healthy foods. Certain genes may also make us less likely to engage in physical activity (UK Cancer Research, 2009).

ENVIRONMENT VERSUS GENETICS

While approximately 25% of the variation among people in body fat levels is determined by genetic factors, studies have shown that cultural or environmental factors are a bigger influence, accounting for 30% (Bouchard et al., 1988 cited in Heyward, 2006).

Why is this the case? Over the past 30 years our environment has increasingly promoted the consumption of energy-dense food, as well as a reliance on technology that decreases the level of physical activity that we undertake (Heyward, 2006).

Although understanding how our genes influence obesity is critical in trying to understand the current obesity epidemic, it is important to remember that genetic traits alone do not mean that obesity is inevitable. Our lifestyle is critical when it comes to determining how fat we are, regardless of our genetic traits (Lifespan, 2012).

Research suggests it may be possible to minimise genetic risk by changing our eating patterns and adopting other healthy lifestyle habits, such as regular physical activity (Lifespan, 2012). In other words, it is possible to be relatively lean through a healthy diet and physical activity, even if you have a genetic predisposition to obesity. On the other hand, however, it is possible to become obese due to lifestyle, even without a genetic predisposition.

A MATTER OF BALANCE

Although various factors may influence a person's body fat levels, as we've discussed, the fundamental cause for people becoming overweight and obese is energy imbalance (McArdle et al., 2010; Heyward, 2006; UK Cancer Research, 2009; WHO, 2012).

If the energy from the food we consume equals the energy we expend, our body fat stores remain unchanged. This is known as energy balance. However, when our energy intake is greater than the amount of energy we expend or burn off, this creates an energy imbalance where the excess energy will be stored as fat (WHO, 2012). One kilogram of fat is approximately 7,000kcal of unused energy.

Globally, there has been an increased intake of energy-dense foods that are high in fat, salt and sugars, but low in vitamins, minerals and other micronutrients, which not only lack sufficient nutrients for optimal health but can also lead to increases in body fat (WHO, 2012).

The increased consumption of high-calorie food has been accompanied by a decrease in energy expenditure, due to factors including the increasingly sedentary nature of many forms of work; changing modes of transport; the use of labour-saving devices and inactive leisure activities such as computer games (WHO, 2012; House of Commons, 2004).

Just a small energy imbalance can lead to a significant increase in body fat over time. If your energy intake exceeds expenditure by just 100kcal per day – which is about the same amount of calories contained in a regular size skinny latte coffee – over the course of a year this could lead to an increase in body fat of 4.7kg (10.3lb). On the other hand, if you reduce your daily food intake by 100 calories per day and increase your energy expenditure by 100 calories – perhaps by walking or jogging an extra mile a day – your energy expenditure over the course of a year would equal the amount of energy in 9.5kg (21lb) of fat (McArdle et al., 2010).

ENERGY EXPENDITURE EXPLAINED

Our total daily energy expenditure is influenced by three main factors:

- Resting energy expenditure
- Physical activity excess
- The thermic effect of eating

(McArdle et al., 2010)

Resting energy expenditure, or resting metabolic rate (RMR), accounts for approximately 50-75% of the total daily energy expenditure of the average person (McArdle et al., 2010).

Here's a quick calculation you can do to work out how many calories you need just to support your body's energy requirements at rest. You might be surprised by the result.

QUICK ESTIMATE OF RESTING METABOLIC RATE (RMR)

Men: RMR kcal/day = body weight (BW) in kilograms (kg) x 24.2
Women: RMR kcal/day = BW (kg) x 22

(Heyward, 2006)

For example, if you were a male weighing 100kg you would have an estimated RMR of 2,420 calories per day (100 x 24.2 = 2,420 kcal/day)

To put this into perspective, you would need to eat 2,420 calories just to maintain your body's essential functions while you are resting.

A common misconception is that obese people have lower resting metabolic rates than those of normal weight people. However, as RMR is related to body size and surface area, taller, heavier people have a higher

RMR than shorter, lighter people. Obese people often have a considerable amount of muscle mass because they have to carry more weight around (McArdle et al., 1996; Wilmore and Costill, 2004). Ageing tends to lower our resting metabolic rate, as it typically decreases by 2-5% per decade after the age of 40 (Heyward, 2006).

PHYSICAL ACTIVITY AND ENERGY EXPENDITURE

Physical activity is the most variable component of daily energy expenditure and has by far the greatest effect. For example, an athlete may nearly double his or her daily energy output, expending 2000kcals, as a result of 3-4 hours of hard training, while a sedentary person may expend as little as 100kcal in a whole day (Wilmore et al., 2008). Typically, physical activity accounts for approximately 15-30% of our daily energy expenditure. It is essential for achieving and maintaining healthy body fat levels, as it reduces the 'normal' pattern of fat gain in adulthood and reduces the tendency to regain body fat after weight loss (McArdle et al., 2010).

Even after we have finished exercise our metabolism remains elevated for some time. This is referred to as excess post-exercise oxygen consumption or 'after burn'. Typically, 15kcals are spent during recovery for every 100kcal spent during exercise (Wilmore and Costill, 2004).

YOU ARE WHAT YOU EAT: DIETARY THERMOGENESIS

Some of the energy we consume is used to digest, absorb, metabolise and store food in the body (McArdle et al., 2010). This is referred to as dietary thermogenesis or the thermic effect of food. Although there can be considerable variation between individuals, the thermic effect of food accounts for 10-30% of the calories we consume, depending on the quantity and composition of the food. We tend to burn more calories after consuming carbohydrate and protein, for example, compared to fat (McArdle et al., 2010).

In summary, regardless of the various factors that influence our levels of body fat, the fundamental cause of overweight and obesity is energy imbalance.

We cannot alter our genes and it is very difficult to control our environment, but we can make lifestyle choices, such as eating healthily and being physically active, which will help us to achieve and maintain healthy body fat levels.

In the next chapter, we will look at how to plan your fat loss programme. and you use your fridge full of treats to help relax and unwind.

4

PLANNING YOUR FAT LOSS PROGRAMME

In order to successfully achieve and maintain healthy body fat levels it is essential that you first understand what a healthy level of body fat is for you, as well as the safest and most effective way to achieve it. Of course, people often look to those in the media spotlight as role models when it comes to body shape and size. However, regardless of the achievements for which they are famous, those actors, sports stars, musicians and household names are not always good role models in terms of body fat levels. They could, for instance, be unhealthily low as a result of their professional sporting lifestyle or simply be unrealistic or unhealthy for the average person.

A study estimated that models and actresses in the 1990s had 10-15% body fat, while the average body fat for a healthy woman today, for good health, is considered to be 20-32% (ACSM, 2010). Athletes can often have even lower levels of body fat. For example, female runners typically have body fat levels of 8-15% (Wilmore et al., 2008). Similarly, male marathon runners can be as low as 3.3% (McArdle et al., 2010), while a level of 10-22% is generally recommended in men for good health (ACSM, 2010; Esmat, 2012).

HOW MUCH FAT DO I NEED TO LOSE?

This is, of course, probably the most important question in this book. However, it is in itself a carefully worded question as the crucial word is 'need' and not 'want'. Indeed, there could be a significant difference between the fat you want to lose and the fat you actually need to lose. So the real question is actually: how much fat, if any, do you need to lose to be healthy? The health risks associated with excessive body fat levels are well acknowledged, such as an increased risk of developing serious health problems including coronary artery disease, hypertension, type 2 diabetes and certain types of cancer (ACSM, 2010).

On the other hand, people with too little body fat tend to be malnourished and have a relatively higher risk of osteoporosis, bone fractures, muscle wasting, abnormal heart rhythms and sudden death, as well as kidney and reproductive disorders (Heyward and Stolarzyck, 1996; Hanlon, 1995).
The first step in designing your fat loss programme is therefore to ascertain where you should be between these two extremes. Here's how you can find out.

WAIST CIRCUMFERENCE

One way we tend to notice if we have put on body fat is by the way our clothes fit, particularly around the waist. A simple waist measurement is, therefore, probably the easiest way to find out if you need to lose some body fat.

Where we carry our body fat, regardless of how much total body fat we have, is generally acknowledged as an important predictor of the health risks associated with obesity. As we saw in Chapter Two, those of us with an apple body shape will see most of our body fat deposited on our abdomens and, consequently, we'll be at greater risk of developing a number of different health problems such as hypertension, type 2 diabetes and coronary heart disease. Those of us with a pear body shape, meanwhile, will see most of our body fat deposited on our hips and thighs (Heyward, 2006; Mayo Clinic, 2011) and we'll be less at risk of the health problems associated with an apple shape.

As a general guideline, you have a higher risk of health problems if you are a man and your waist size is more than 94cm (37 inches) or if you are a woman and your waist is more than 80cm (31.5 inches) (NHS, 2012).

The risk of health problems is even higher for men if their waist size is more than 102cm (40 inches) and for women if their waist more than 88cm (34.5 inches) (NHS, 2012; ACSM, 2010).

HOW TO MEASURE YOUR WAIST PROPERLY

- Stand with your feet together and your abdomen relaxed
- Find the bottom of your ribs and the top of your hips
- Breathe out naturally
- Wrap a tape measure around your waist, midway between these points, without compressing the fat
- Ensure that the tape measure is horizontal
- Record the measurement to the nearest centimetre

(Adapted from ACSM, 2006; NHS, 2012)

BODY MASS INDEX (BMI)

Body Mass Index, or BMI, is an often quoted term with which you may be familiar. It is simply a mathematical formula to ascertain a person's weight relative to their height and is calculated by dividing your body weight in kilograms by your height in metres squared (w/ht^2).

For example, if you weigh 75kg and are 1.78m tall then you would have a BMI of 23.7.

BMI is commonly used to classify people as underweight, normal, overweight and obese.

The NHS offers a BMI calculator on its website:

http://www.nhs.uk/Livewell/loseweight/Pages/BodyMassIndex.aspx

It also classifies 'underweight' as those with a BMI below 18.5; 'healthy weight' as those with a BMI between 18.5-24.9; 'above the ideal range' as those with a BMI of 25 or more and 'obese' as those with a BMI of 30 or more.

BMI: ADVANTAGES AND LIMITATIONS

The main advantages of BMI are that it is inexpensive, simple and quick. It is useful as a population-level measure of overweight and obesity as it is the same for both sexes and for all ages of adults (WHO, 2012).

However, it should be considered a rough guide because it may not correspond to the same degree of fatness in different individuals. It overestimates the fatness of people that are very muscular, such as body builders, and can underestimate fatness in people who have lost muscle mass, such as the elderly (Heyward and Stolarczyk, 1996). Also, it does not adequately reflect changes in fat and muscle mass that occur as a result of weight loss (ACSM, 2010).

People who are very short (under 1.5m) may have a high BMI that does not reflect their true body fat levels, as would people suffering from excessive accumulation of fluid in the tissues of the body (Heyward and Stolarczyk, 1996).

Central YMCA (authors of APPG report on body image, 2012), meanwhile, believes that BMI should be revised. The measure was developed in the 1830s to compare large swathes of populations and while Central YMCA understands that it is a useful indicator at epidemiological levels, it believes that BMI is a blunt and inaccurate measure of someone's health. For example, BMI says nothing about body composition, such as level of muscularity or bone density. It also doesn't give an indication of where fat is distributed within the body, i.e. visceral or subcutaneous.

The APPG on Body Image concluded that BMI should be reviewed, and potentially revised to take account of differences in genders, age groups and ethnicities. It also believes that BMI should be used in collaboration with other health indicators, such as waist circumference or measure of subjective wellbeing, to indicate a person's overall health more accurately.

BODY COMPOSITION

Most people tend to judge their level of fatness by what their bathroom scales tell them; however this can be very misleading. With regard to overall health, weight is not as important as the composition of our bodies, which shows the relative proportions of fat and lean mass in our body and is expressed as a percentage of our body weight (Esmat, 2012).

For example, a typical sedentary woman may gain 14kg (30lb) in weight between the ages of 20 and 50. However, she is likely to have gained 20kg (45Ib) of fat and lost 7kg (15Ib) of muscle, increasing her percentage of fat from 23% to 47% (Wescott, 2003), which would not show up on her bathroom scales.

While we have two types of fat – essential fat and nonessential, or storage, fat – the second component of body composition, lean mass or fat-free mass, refers to your muscle, bones, tissues and organs.

Although there appears to be no universally accepted norm for the amount of body fat a person should have, but it is generally accepted that a range of 10-22% for men and 20-32% for women is considered satisfactory for good health (ACSM, 2010; Esmat, 2012).

There are a number of different methods available to provide us with an assessment of our level of body fat, ranging in complexity, accuracy and expense from tape measures, skinfold callipers and bioelectrical impedance to underwater weighing and MRI scans.

DEFINING YOUR WEIGHT LOSS GOAL (AT A HEALTHY LEVEL OF BODY FAT)

If you are able to assess your body fat percentage, you can use this information and a calculator to find out what your body weight should be at a healthier level of body fat. For example, if you are female and weigh 72kg with 38% body fat and you wish to reduce your body fat to a healthier 28%, you would calculate your desirable body weight at that fat percentage in the following way:

- Determine your fat weight by multiplying your body weight by your percentage body fat (72 x 0.38 = 27.36kg)
- Find your fat-free weight by subtracting your fat weight from your total weight (72 - 27.36kg = 44.64 kg)
- Calculate your goal fat-free mass by subtracting your goal body fat from 100% (100-28% = 72% fat-free mass)
- Find your body weight goal by dividing your current fat-free mass by your new fat-free mass goal (44.64/ 0.72 = 62kg)
- Determine your weight loss goal by subtracting your body weight goal from your current weight (72 - 62kg = 10kg)

(Hanlon, 1995; McArdle, 2010)

So in this example you would need to lose 10kg of fat to achieve your target body fat percentage of 28%.

HOW MUCH SHOULD I AIM TO LOSE INITIALLY?

Unless a health care professional suggests otherwise, your fat loss goal should be to reduce your body weight by 5-15%, regardless of how much weight you ultimately need to lose. Setting weight loss targets beyond 5-15% often gives people unrealistic and potentially unachievable targets (McArdle et al., 2010). As a general guideline, rate of weight loss should be 5-10% of initial body weight over a three to six month period (ACSM,

2010).

Even a small amount of fat loss can improve your health. Losing as little as 3% has been associated with favourable changes in chronic disease risk factors (Donnelly et al., 2009). For example, a 10kg weight loss has been shown to provide:

1. 20% reduction in total mortality
2. 30% reduction in diabetes-related deaths
3. 40% reduction in obesity-related cancers
4. 10mm Hg reduction in systolic blood pressure
5. 20 mmHg reduction in diastolic blood pressure
6. 50% reduction in fasting glucose
7. 10% reduction in total cholesterol
8. 8% increase in so-called 'good cholesterol' or HDL
9. 30% reduction in triglycerides

(SIGN, 1996)

How do we achieve this?

If our energy intake from food and drink is less than the energy we expend through activity, our body will draw on its own fat stores for energy. Research shows that most adults eat and drink more than they need, and think that they are more physically active than they actually are (NHS, 2010). A healthy fat loss programme creates a negative energy balance that will allow the body to use up more fat stores than fat-free mass, which includes muscle.

If energy intake is reduced slowly without too severe a restriction, approximately 75% of the energy shortfall will come from fat and the remaining 25% from fat-free mass (McKardle, 1996).

How fast should we reduce our fat stores?

Unless a health care professional suggests otherwise, and regardless of your total fat loss goal, you should only aim to lose 0.5 to 1kg (1 to 2.2Ib) per week (ACSM, 2010; Heyward, 2006; McArdle et al., 2010).

A daily energy deficit of 500 to 1,000kcals produces a weekly shortfall of 3,500 to 7,000kcal, which equates to a weight loss of 0.5kg (1.1Ib) to 1kg (2.2Ibs) per week. Your daily energy deficit should not exceed 1,000kcal, as this can lead to a greater loss of muscle. So if a person needs to lose 10kg, as in our earlier example, they should allow 10-20 weeks.

It is important that you create only a moderate energy deficit, as it has been shown that energy deficits greater than 700kcal/day, although producing overall greater weight loss, can also result in a loss of muscle (Mayo et al., 2003).

To achieve the desired rate of fat loss we need to reduce our energy intake by approximately 200 to 300kcal per day, the equivalent of 50g of potato crisps, and expend an additional 300kcal per day through physical activity (ACSM, 2010).

In the next chapter, we will look at the most effective way to use exercise and physical activity to help you reduce your body fat levels.

Central YMCA Health and Fitness Guides

5

CREATING YOUR FAT BURNING PROGRAMME

We all know that exercise can play a vital role in helping you to achieve and maintain healthy levels of body fat. Not only does it increase your energy expenditure, it also helps to increase the amount of fat you lose when compared to dieting alone and maintains or reduces the loss of muscle that can result from dieting (Heyward, 2006).

In order to gain from the many benefits of exercise and to maximise its fat burning potential you need to perform the right type and quantity of exercise. However, only about half the number of people trying to reduce their body fat levels use the recommended method of reducing energy intake and increasing activity levels, and only a minority of those perform the recommended amount of activity (Heyward, 2006). Like any other fitness programme, you need to tailor the programme to suit your needs and abilities. For example, if a person is new to exercise and very overweight their initial programme will be different from the programme of a fit, active person who just wishes to drop a few pounds.

DO I NEED TO GO TO THE GYM?

The short answer to this question is no.

Although the terms 'exercise' and 'physical activity' are often used interchangeably, they actually have slightly different meanings.

Exercise is a type of physical activity, which is defined as 'planned, structured and repetitive bodily movement done to improve or maintain one or more components of physical fitness, such as strength'.

Physical activity, meanwhile, can be defined as 'any bodily movement that is produced by skeletal muscle and that substantially increases energy expenditure'. The more vigorous activities of daily living such as raking the lawn and vacuuming would be classified as physical activity (ACSM, 2010). Remember, we are trying to create an energy deficit, so a good approach for many individuals to obtain the recommended level of physical activity is to incorporate more incidental and leisure-time activity into their daily routine (Saris et al., 2003).

For example, if a person weighs 100kg and wants to burn 300 to 500kcal they could either walk at a speed of 4km/hr for 1-1.5 hours or dig the garden for approximately 40 minutes. There are plenty of calorie expenditure tables available online to help you work out your energy expenditure.

WHAT TYPE OF EXERCISE DO I NEED TO DO?

Aerobic activities such as walking, running, cycling and rowing should make up the majority of your exercise programme. Resistance training should also be included.

PLANNING YOUR AEROBIC EXERCISE PRESCRIPTION

How often do I need to do it? You will need to exercise five days per week or more to maximise energy expenditure and achieve significant fat loss (ACSM, 2010).

How hard do I need to work? Depending on your fitness level, you should work from moderate to vigorous intensity.

Moderate intensity is defined as the level of exertion that noticeably increases your heart rate and breathing. If you use heart rate reserve (HRR)* to calculate your training heart rates this equates to 40 to 60%. Alternatively, you may use rate of perceived exertion (RPE) to monitor exercise intensity. If so, you should work to 'moderate' 3 on the 0-10 RPE scale.

Vigorous intensity is defined as a level of exertion that substantially increases your heart rate and breathing. This equates to a 50 to 75% of heart rate reserve and a RPE of 'moderate to hard' 5 or 6 on the 0-10 RPE scale (ACSM, 2010).

Typically, you should begin by working at a moderate intensity and eventually, if appropriate, progress to vigorous intensity. This may provide you with increased health and fitness benefits (ACSM 2010) and will allow you to expend the required amount of energy in a shorter time, when compared to moderate intensity exercise.

*If you are unfamiliar with calculating your heart rate reserve, there a number of online resources available, including:

http://www.briancalkins.com/HeartRate.htm

http://www.sportfit.com/sportfitglossary/energetics_aerobic_krvnn.html

How many minutes do I need to exercise?

The commonly quoted guideline of 30 minutes of physical activity a day expends approximately 200kcal, which is slightly more than half of the energy expenditure required for significant fat loss (ACSM, 2010). Ideally, you should perform 30 to 60 minutes per day, or two sessions of 20 to 30 minutes to a total of 150 minutes per week, progressing to 300 minutes per week of moderate physical activity. Alternatively, you could look to tally up 150 minutes of vigorous physical activity, or an equivalent of moderate and vigorous physical activity, per week (ACSM, 2010; Donnelley et al., 2009).

It may be necessary for some very overweight people to progress to 60 to 90 minutes of exercise daily if they wish to lose a significant amount of fat and maintain their weight (ACSM, 2010; Donnelley et al., 2009).

You don't have to do all of this exercise in one continuous workout; you can break it down into blocks of intermittent exercise of at least 10 minutes' duration each throughout the day (Donnelly et al., 2009).

What is the best mode of exercise?

The recommended type or mode of exercise is that of large muscle aerobic activities, such as walking, cycling, rowing, water aerobics, jogging and so on (ACSM, 2010).

However, you have to enjoy what you're doing, so select a mode of exercise that you prefer and which accommodates your personal needs and abilities.

For example, due to the increased risk of orthopaedic injury in obese people, low impact activities such as walking are preferable to high impact activities such as running. For some very large or deconditioned people, non-weight-bearing activities, such as cycling, may be more appropriate (Wallace and Ray, 2009).

Studies comparing different modes of exercise, such as cycling, jogging and walking tend to show that they are equally effective in reducing body fat stores (Heyward, 2006; McArdle et al., 2010).

Running, however, is usually most effective at maximising energy expenditure during continuous exercise, providing you have no injuries or health problems which would make it inappropriate (McArdle et al., 2010). You might like to spread your exercise time between several different modes, such as 10 minutes on the bike, rower and treadmill to add some variety to your programme.

A common mistake when comparing the fat burning effectiveness of different modes of exercise is just to compare activities over the same period. For example, you will burn more kcal in half an hour of running when compared to walking for the same period; you could burn the same amount of energy walking, you'll just need to walk for longer.

HOW MANY CALORIES SHOULD I AIM TO BURN?

You should aim to burn approximately 2,000kcal/week or more (ACSM, 2010; Wallace and Ray, 2009; Donnelly et al., 2009). Modern exercise equipment can give you a reasonable indication of your calorie energy expenditure.

HOW DO I START?

If you are new to this no one expects you to start with 90 minutes per day of vigorous exercise. You should aim to start slowly and progress gradually (McArdle et al., 2010). You could start, for example, with 20 to 30 minutes of moderate intensity, or less, perhaps broken down into 10 minute blocks. Then you can work towards combining these blocks into one session.

An increase in duration of approximately 5 to 10% per week is generally appropriate. For example, in Week 1 you could perform a total of 20 minutes of low intensity exercise per session and then increase this time by approximately 2 to 3 minutes per week until you can perform 60 minutes by Weeks 11 or 12. At this point you may want to cut the duration to 45 minutes and increase the intensity to vigorous. You can then up the duration by 5 to 10% per week until you reach the desired duration at the higher intensity.

The reason for the initial focus on duration is not that low intensity exercise is more effective than higher intensity exercise for fat burning, it is because people carrying a lot of body fat are generally poorly conditioned, and are at an increased risk of cardiovascular disease. They may also have had poor experiences with exercise, so to initiate the programme too aggressively may decrease their adherence and increase their risk of injury (ACSM, 2006: McArdle et al., 2010).

Never increase duration and intensity in the same session. You can't expect to work longer *and* harder.

WHY DO WE NEED TO DO SO MUCH?

Research has shown moderate-intensity physical activity between 150 and 250 minutes per week to be effective to prevent weight gain but will provide only modest fat loss. However, greater amounts of physical activity (>250 minutes per week) have been associated with clinically significant fat loss (Donnelly et al., 2009).

It is important to remember that the guidelines for the time spent exercising also include the time spent performing resistance training, but your primary type of exercise should be aerobic.

GETTING THE MOST BANG FOR YOUR BUCK: MAXIMISING ENERGY EXPENDITURE

For some people, a moderate intensity programme is all they wish to do or are able to do, so progression to higher intensity work would not be appropriate. Additionally, high intensity exercise is associated with poorer adherence (ACSM, 2006). However, you may not have the time or the inclination to do five or more long training sessions per week, so you need to be able to maximise your energy expenditure in other ways.

Set pace: This involves deciding the duration of the exercise session, for example 30 minutes, and then setting the intensity as high as possible to ensure that fatigue occurs gradually over 30 minutes. As your fitness improves, the exercise can be sustained at a higher intensity and more energy will be expended in the 30 minute period (Wilmore and Costill, 2004). Remember, the idea is not to exercise to exhaustion.

Interval training: This comprises a repeated series of high intensity workouts interspersed with periods of light activity. It is based on the concept that more work can be performed at higher exercise intensities with less fatigue than experienced with continuous training (Brooks, 1998). This form of training can be used to develop speed, and aerobic and anaerobic power, depending on the protocol you use.

Aerobic interval training provides a good introduction to more high intensity training. Follow these guidelines:

How hard? Generally an intensity of 80 to 85% HRR or equivalent RPE of 'somewhat hard to very hard' is used for the work intervals, with the recovery intervals being at around 50% of HRR and RPE 'light' (Brooks, 1998). A lower intensity of 75% of HRR for the work interval may be more appropriate for less well conditioned people.

How long? As a general guideline, long aerobic intervals tend be 3 to 8 minutes with similar duration active recovery between intervals (Sleamaker and Browning, 1996). This provides an effort to recovery ratio of 1:1. You can begin with intervals as short as two minutes and then progress to longer durations. You can also progress to having a recovery period only half the length of the work interval (Sleamaker and Browning, 1996).

How many? The number of intervals you perform depends on how much time you have available and how fit you are. Generally, 5 to 10 work–recovery intervals would be performed in a session (Sleamaker and Browning 1996; Wilmore and Costill, 2004).

HIGH INTENSITY INTERVAL TRAINING: THE WAY AHEAD FOR FAT BURNING?

In the last few years you may have come across reports in the media regarding the use of high intensity interval training (HIIT) for fat loss. This attention has resulted from a number of studies suggesting that HIIT may not only be more time efficient than other forms of exercise, but also more effective at reducing body fat levels (Irving et al., 2008; King et al., 2001; Tremblay et al., 1994; Boutcher, 2011).

The results of the studies have shown that when the participants expended exactly the same amount of energy performing steady state, moderate intensity cardiovascular exercise and HIIT, the HIIT produced greater reductions in body fat. In one study the average estimated total energy cost of the moderate exercise was 48% greater than the energy expenditure for the HIIT programme. However, despite its lower energy cost, the HIIT programme produced nine-fold greater reduction in subcutaneous fat compared with the moderate intensity exercise when the exercise volume was taken into account (Tremblay et al., 1994).

HIIT may also be more effective for reducing total abdominal fat than lower intensity exercise (Irving et al., 2008) and has also been shown to increase both aerobic and anaerobic fitness significantly, and to provide health benefits such as a reduction in insulin resistance (Boutcher, 2011).

Various interval formats have been used in the studies (Boutcher, 2011). For example, 30 seconds of all-out sprint cycling 4 to 6 times, separated by 4 minutes of recovery, which equates to approximately 3 to 4 minutes of exercise per session.

Other less demanding protocols have included an eight-second cycle sprint followed by 12 seconds of low intensity cycling for a period of 20 minutes (Trapp et al., 2008), a 15-second cycle sprint followed by 15 seconds of low intensity cycling for a period of 20 minutes (Whyte et al., 2010), and a two-minute cycle at 95% of VO2max alternating with three minutes at 25% of VO2max (King et al., 2001).

However, before you rush off and start sprint training it is important to note that HIIT can be extremely demanding and you may have to tolerate significant discomfort in the process. Consequently, high intensity training should be progressed to gradually and is not suitable for people with an increased risk of cardiovascular disease, pre-existing disease or orthopaedic conditions (ACSM, 2006). If you are at all unsure, seek the advice of a health professional.

THE TRUTH ABOUT THE FAT BURNING ZONE

You may have heard that the most effective way to reduce body fat levels is to exercise in the 'fat burning zone'. This concept has come about due to a misunderstanding regarding the optimal exercise intensity at which your body uses a greater percentage of fat as fuel and how your body reduces its body fat stores with exercise.

In short, at lower exercise intensities your body uses a greater percentage of fat as fuel than at higher intensities. However, the amount of body fat you lose due to exercise is determined by the total kcal expenditure and not by the fuel source. High intensity interval training is typically performed at a higher intensity than the fat burning zone, but as we saw in the earlier example has been shown to be more effective at reducing body fat stores than lower intensity exercise.

MIX AND MATCH TO ADD VARIETY

You can use a variety of different types of aerobic exercise sessions in your fat burning programme.
For example, you may choose to do a long workout of 60 to 90 minutes at a moderate intensity. On another day you may try an aerobic interval session or perhaps a set pace session. As your fitness increases you might attempt some high intensity intervals. Remember, the important thing is to create the required energy deficit for you in a safe and enjoyable way.

RESISTANCE TRAINING

Resistance training is now generally viewed as a vital aide to aerobic exercise. Indeed, a combination of the two has been shown to produce greater reductions in body fat compared with aerobic exercise alone (Brochu et al., 2009).

Studies comparing resistance training with aerobic endurance training suggest that resistance training has uniquely beneficial effects on body composition as it decreases body fat while increasing muscle. Aerobic endurance training, meanwhile, decreases fat levels with no change in muscle. As muscle is more metabolically active than fat, the increases in muscle will increase your resting daily expenditure (McArdle et al., 2010).

On average, previously sedentary clients can replace approximately three pounds of muscle after about three months of regular resistance training, which can result in an approximate increase in RMR of 7% (Westcott and Guy, 1996 cited in Wescott, 2003).

Resistance training can also be good for calorie burning as circuit resistance training has been shown to burn 9kcal per minute. It can also help you to keep burning extra calories long after your training session has finished. You may have come across the term 'metabolic training' recently in the fitness press. Although definitions vary, it generally refers to the use of high intensity resistance training to stimulate your metabolism for considerable periods after your training session. Although the calories burned during exercise are generally considered the most important factor in total exercise energy expenditure (McArdle et al., 2010), the energy expended above resting values after exercise, which is known as excess post-exercise oxygen consumption or 'after burn', still contribute to your fat loss.

For example, one study, which involved participants performing 31 minutes of resistance training consisting of four circuits of 10 repetitions to failure of bench press, power cleans and squats, found that it significantly increased the participants' post-exercise oxygen consumption for 38 hours after the training session (Schuenke et al., 2002). So for 38 hours after their training session the participants' bodies were constantly working to reduce their fat stores.

There does not appear to be specific resistance training guidelines for fat loss; however, the guidelines for muscular fitness for health provide a good basis for a suitable resistance training programme as they will help to increase muscle mass.

Mentioning the words 'increase muscle' can cause some people, particularly women, to panic as they imagine themselves suddenly becoming too bulky. However, this is not likely to happen as muscle is more dense than fat. Indeed, you may lose several pounds of fat and gain several pounds of muscle, but appear slimmer.

What sort of equipment should I use?

You can use almost any form of resistance equipment such as free weights, resistance machines or resistance bands. However, some people's size may affect their ability to access certain equipment and limit their range of motion.

How often should I do resistance training?

If you train your whole body in a single session, you should perform two to three times per week on non-consecutive days to allow at least 48 hours recovery between training sessions (ACSM, 2010).

Intensity, sets and reps

The aim of the programme is to maintain or increase muscle mass. Consequently, an 8-12 repetition range is most appropriate.

You should select a resistance that allows you to perform two to four sets of 8-12 repetitions per muscle group to the point of approximate momentary muscular fatigue (ACSM, 2010). This is the point that momentary failure occurs in the concentric phase of an exercise. For example, when you raise the bar in a biceps curl, preventing another rep being performed with good form in that set.

Older people and very deconditioned individuals should perform one or more sets of 10-15 reps at a 'moderate' level of RPE. They can progress up to the 8-12 reps range after a period of adaptation (ACSM, 2010).

HOW DO I KNOW WHEN TO INCREASE THE RESISTANCE?

There are various methods that can be used to increase resistance. A conservative method is the two-for-two rule: If you can perform two or more repetitions over your repetition goal in the last set in two consecutive workouts, you should increase the resistance in the next training session (Brooks, 1998).

HOW MANY EXERCISES SHOULD I DO?

If you are training your whole body in a single session, you should aim for 8 to 10 exercises that target all the major muscle groups, that is legs, chest, back, shoulders and so on (ACSM, 2010).

WHICH EXERCISES ARE BEST?

Multi-joint exercises such as squats, bench press, rows, dead lifts and cleans are preferred because the involvement of several muscle groups makes them time efficient (ACSM, 2010) and they typically burn more kcal than isolation exercises, such as flyes. Additionally, they tend to be more functional as many activities of everyday living involve multi-joint movements.

If possible, try to perform different exercises for each muscle group every two to three sessions to ensure even development and reduce the chances of overuse injury (ACSM, 2006). For example, you may perform lateral pull-downs for a couple of workouts and then replace these with cable rows.

HOW QUICKLY SHOULD I PERFORM THE EXERCISES?

A slow to moderate tempo is generally recommended (Clark and Corn, 2001). For example, when performing the bench press exercise, you may take approximately four seconds to lower the bar, pause for a couple of seconds and then take two seconds to raise the bar.

HOW LONG SHOULD I REST BETWEEN SETS?

You need to allow adequate recovery between sets to enable the next one to be performed with correct form. Typically, a recovery of one to two minutes is recommended (Baechle and Earle, 2000) although you may initially require a little longer. Try to complete the exercise session within one hour, as longer sessions are associated with higher dropout rates (ACSM, 2006).

Here's an example of a typical resistance training programme:

EXERCISE	SETS
Squats	2 - 4
Barbell bench press	2 - 4
Romanian deadlift	2 - 4
Cable row	2 - 4
Dumbbell shoulder press	2 - 4
Biceps curl	2 - 4
Triceps curl	2 - 4
Calf-raise	2 - 4

Plus core exercises

OPTIMISING THE CALORIE BURNING POTENTIAL OF YOUR RESISTANCE TRAINING

There are a number of ways you can increase the energy expenditure of your resistance training sessions, including:

Vary the training programme: As your body adapts to training stimulus it no longer requires as much energy to perform the work. This phenomenon is known as accommodation. Consequently, you should change your training programme regularly by using different exercises, varying the intensity, exercise order, etc. If you are new to exercise and are training two to three times per week it will take approximately one to three months for your body to adapt to the imposed demands of the training programme (Clarke and Corn, 2001).

Use single limb exercises where appropriate: These require greater energy expenditure than exercises that involve both limbs. For example, performing a set of single arm dumbbell chest presses for each arm will burn more calories than a set of barbell chest presses (Clarke and Corn, 2001).

As you get fitter you can try reducing the rest periods between sets, which results in greater energy expenditure (Clarke and Corn, 2001).

COMBINED SESSIONS

You may choose to perform your resistance training and aerobic training on separate days. However, this is not always possible or preferable. Consequently, it may be necessary for you to perform both the aerobic and resistance training in the same session. So in this instance you could perform the resistance training followed by the aerobic exercise, or vice versa. Alternatively, you could intersperse periods of aerobic exercise with resistance training. This can make your sessions more interesting and allow you to accumulate a greater amount of high intensity aerobic exercise than you may be able to sustain for a single, longer period.

Here are a couple of examples:

EXAMPLE 1 (60-70 MINUTES)

- Warm up (5-10 minutes) low-to-moderate CV
- 10 minutes moderate-to-high intensity CV
- 30 minutes of resistance training performed either in the standard resistance training sets format, or in a circuit, where one set of each exercise is completed before returning to the first exercise for the second set and so on. The circuit format with minimal recoveries can be a very time efficient method of kcal expenditure, with reports of expenditures of 200kcal for 15 minutes of activity (Anderson, 2004).
- 10 minutes of moderate-to-high intensity CV
- Cool down (5-10) minutes low-to-moderate CV

EXAMPLE 2 (60 MINUTES)

- 5 minute CV warm up
- 10 minutes circuit resistance training
- 10 minutes moderate-to-high intensity CV
- 10 minutes circuit resistance training
- 10minutes moderate-to-high intensity CV
- 10 minutes circuit resistance training
- 5 minute CV cool down

If you are new to exercise you can adapt the workouts by reducing both the volume and intensity of the exercise. For example, you may perform only low-to-moderate aerobic exercise and reduce the resistance exercise to one set or circuit.

GENERAL TRAINING TIPS

Have flexible rather than rigid exercise goals. Although the recommended exercise guidelines are important don't be put off if you can't adhere to them as any activity is better than nothing (ACSM, 2000).

Be aware that people carrying a lot of body fat are at risk of hyperthermia (elevated body temperature) (Wallace and Ray, 2009). To help reduce the risk of heat illness ensure you drink sufficient fluids, wear appropriate clothing, avoid exercising at the hottest part of the day and exercise in a cool environment such as a shady, breezy site, or indoors where the temperature can be controlled (ACSM, 2010; Wilmore et al., 2008).

Find any excuse to expend a calorie. Try to 'generalise' your exercise habit from the gym to other environments, such as parking the car further from the shops, having walk breaks at work, using stairs rather than a lift and so on (ACSM, 2000).

Set long- and short-term goals. For example, if your long-term goal is to lose 10kg this could be broken down to a short-term goal of 0.5 kg per week.

Try to get some social support. The support of family and friends can help you to stick to your fat loss programme. Try to find a compatible exercise partner who has the same goals as you and who can encourage and support you (ACSM, 2000).

6

IN CONCLUSION

Although the theory of fat loss is very simple – expend more energy than you consume – the high rates of failure among people to achieve and maintain healthy body fat levels show us just how difficult it can be in practice.

Typically, participants in supervised fat-loss programmes lose about 8 to 12% of their original body weight (McArdle et al., 2010). However, the average weight regain is approximately 33 to 50% of initial weight loss within a year of finishing the programme (ACSM, 2010).

Attempts to reduce body fat tend to be more successful when losses are only 0.45 to 0.9kg (1-2Ib) per week and when dietary restriction (300-500 fewer kcal per day) is combined with moderate exercise. This combination minimises the loss of fat-free mass and maximises fat loss (Wilmore et al., 2008).

You are also more likely to be successful in reducing and maintaining your body fat stores at a healthy level if you:

- Carry your fat on your upper body
- Are only slightly or moderately obese
- Have no history of repeatedly losing and regaining weight
- Became obese as an adult
- Have a strong desire to reduce your body fat levels (Wallace and Ray, 2009)

- Maintain an exercise programme, as the maintenance of exercise may be one of the best predictors of long-term weight maintenance (ACSM, 2001)

Your fat loss goals should be based on what is best for your health, not an unhealthy or unrealistic image in the media, and the way you achieve them should be guided by science not fad and fashion.

Remember, once you have achieved your fat loss goal you need to continue with good dietary practice and physical activity indefinitely in order to maintain it.

Good luck.

7

REFERENCES AND FURTHER INFORMATION

REFERENCES: CHAPTER 1

American College of Sports Medicine (2006) *The ACSM's Guidelines for Exercising Testing and Prescription 7th Edition*, Lippincott, Williams and Wilkins, Philadelphia, PA

British Medical Association (2000) *Eating Disorders, Body Image and the Media*, Wiley-Blackwell, London

Disordered Eating (2011) Eating Disorders Statistics [online] Available at: http://www.disordered-eating.co.uk/eating-disorders-statistics/eating-disorders-statistics-uk.html. Accessed 10th November 2012

Heyward, V.H. (2006) *Advanced Fitness Assessment and Exercise Prescription 5th Edition*, Human Kinetics, Champaign, IL

McArdle, W.D., Katch, F.I. and Katch, V.L. (2010) *Exercise Physiology: Energy, Nutrition and Human Performance 7th Edition*, Lippincott Williams and Wilkins, Philadelphia, PA

Scarborough, P. et al. (2010) 'Increased energy intake entirely accounts for increase in body weight in women but not in men in the UK between 1986 and 2000', *British Journal of Nutrition*, 105(9), 1399-404

World Health Organization (2008) Overweight and Obesity Fact Sheet

World Health Organization (2012) Overweight and Obesity Fact Sheet No.311

REFERENCES: CHAPTER 2

Heyward, V.H. (1991) *Advanced Fitness Assessment and Exercise Prescription Human Kinetics 2nd Edition,* Human Kinetics, Champaign, IL

Heyward, V.H. (2006) *Advanced Fitness Assessment and Exercise Prescription 5th Edition,* Human Kinetics, Champaign, IL

Mayo Clinic (2011) Belly fat in women: Taking — and keeping — it off [online] Available at: http://www.mayoclinic.com/health/belly-fat/WO00128. Accessed 13th November 2012

McArdle, W.D., Katch, F.I. and Katch, V.L. (1996) *Exercise Physiology: Energy, Nutrition and Human Performance 4th Edition,* Williams and Wilkins Baltimore, MD

McArdle, W.D., Katch, F.I. and Katch, V.L., (2010) *Exercise Physiology: Energy, Nutrition and Human Performance 7th Edition,* Lippincott Williams and Wilkins, Philadelphia, PA

Wilmore, J.H. and Costill, D.L. (2004) *Physiology of Sport and Exercise 3rd Edition,* Human Kinetics, Champaign, IL

Wilmore, J.H., Costill, D.L. and Kennedy W.L. (2008) *Physiology of Sport and Exercise 4th Edition,* Human Kinetics, Champaign, IL

REFERENCES: CHAPTER 3

Church, C. et al. (2010) 'Overexpression of *Fto* leads to increased food intake and results in obesity', *Nature Genetics,* 42, 1086-96

Heyward, V.H. (1991) *Advanced Fitness Assessment and Exercise Prescription 2nd Edition,* Human Kinetics, Champaign, IL

Heyward, V.H. (2006) *Advanced Fitness Assessment and Exercise Prescription 5th Edition,* Human Kinetics, Champaign, IL

House of Commons Health Select Committee (2004) *Obesity: Third report session 2003-2004, Volume 1.* London: TSO

Lifespan (2012, May 23). "'Obesity genes" may influence food choices, eating patterns', *ScienceDaily* [online] Available at: http://www.sciencedaily.com /releases/2012/05/120523114847.htm. Accessed 16th November 2012.

McArdle, W.D., Katch, F.I. and Katch, V.L. (1996) *Exercise Physiology: Energy, Nutrition and Human Performance 4th Edition,* Williams and Wilkins Baltimore, MD

McArdle, W.D., Katch, F.I. and Katch, V.L., (2010) *Exercise Physiology: Energy, Nutrition and Human Performance 7th Edition,* Lippincott Williams and Wilkins, Philadelphia, PA

Sharkey, B.J. (1990) *Physiology of Fitness 3rd Edition,* Human Kinetics, Champaign, IL

Tortora, G.J., Grabowski, S.R. (2003) *Principles of Anatomy and Physiology 10th Edition,* Wiley, Chichester

UK Cancer Research (2009) The causes of obesity - genes, behaviour and the environment [online]. Available at: www.info.cancerresearchuk.org. Accessed 10th January 2011

Wilmore, J.H. and Costill, D.L. (2004) *Physiology of Sport and Exercise 3rd Edition,* Human Kinetics, Champaign, IL

Wilmore, J.H., Costill, D. L. and Kennedy W.L. (2008) *Physiology of Sport and Exercise 4th Edition* Human Kinetics, Champaign, IL

World Health Organization (2012) Overweight and Obesity Fact Sheet No.311

REFERENCES: CHAPTER 4

American College of Sports Medicine (2006) *The ACSM's Guidelines for Exercising Testing and Prescription 7th Edition*, Lippincott, Williams and Wilkins, Philadelphia, PA

American College of Sports Medicine (2010) *The ACSM's Guidelines for Exercising Testing and Prescription 8th Edition*, Lippincott, Williams and Wilkins, Philadelphia, PA

British Medical Association (2000) *Eating Disorders, Body Image and the Media*, Wiley-Blackwell, London

Donnelly, J.E. et al. (2009) 'Appropriate Physical Activity Intervention Strategies for Weight Loss and Prevention of Weight Regain for Adults', *Medicine and Science in Sports and Exercise*, 41(2), 459-71

Esmat, T. (2012) Measuring and Evaluating Body Composition [online] Available at: www.acsm.org/access-public-information/articles/2012/01/12/measuring-and-evaluating-body-composition. Accessed 21st November 2012

Hanlon. T. (1995) *Practical Body Composition*, Human Kinetics, Champaign, IL

Heyward, V.H. (2006) *Advanced Fitness Assessment and Exercise Prescription 5th Edition*, Human Kinetics, Champaign, IL

Heyward V. H. and Stolarczyk, L.M. (1996) *Applied Body Composition*, Human
Kinetics, Champaign, IL

Mayo Clinic (2011) Belly fat in women: Taking — and keeping — it off [online] Available at: http://www.mayoclinic.com/health/belly-fat/WO00128. Accessed 13th November 2012

Mayo, M.J. et al. (2003) 'Exercise-Induced Weight Lose Preferentially Reduces Abdominal Fat', *Medicine Science Sports and Exercise*, 35(2), 207-213

McArdle, W.D., Katch, F.I. And Katch, V.L. (1996) *Exercise Physiology: Energy, Nutrition and Human Performance 4th Edition*, Williams and Wilkins Baltimore, MD

McArdle, W.D., Katch, F.I. and Katch, V.L. (2010) *Exercise Physiology: Energy, Nutrition and Human Performance 7th Edition*, Lippincott Williams and Wilkins, Philadelphia, PA

NHS (2012) Why is my waist size important? [online] Available at: www.nhs.uk/chq/Pages/849.aspx?CategoryID=51&SubCategoryID=165. Accessed 25th November 2012

NHS (2010) Understanding calories [online] Available at: http://www.nhs.uk/Livewell/loseweight/Pages/understanding-calories.aspx. Accessed 25th November 2012

SIGN (1996) Obesity in Scotland: Integrating Prevention with Weight Management.

Sundgot-Borgen, J., Torstveit, M.K. (2004) 'Prevalence of eating disorders in elite athletes is higher than in the general population', *Clinical Journal of Sport Medicine*, 14, 25-32.

Wescott, W.L. (2003) Senior Strength. Fitpro Feb/March

World Health Organization (2012) Overweight and Obesity Fact Sheet No.311

REFERENCES: CHAPTER 5

ACSM (2001) 'Position Stand on the Appropriate Intervention Strategies for Weight Loss and the Prevention of Weight Regain for Adults', *Medicine and Science in Sports and Exercise,* 33(12), 2145-56

American College of Sports Medicine (2000) *The ACSM Guidelines for Exercising Testing and Prescription 6th Edition*, Lippincott, Williams and Wilkins, Philadelphia, PA

American College of Sports Medicine (2006) *The ACSM's Guidelines for Exercising Testing and Prescription 7th Edition*, Lippincott, Williams and Wilkins, Philadelphia, PA

American College of Sports Medicine (2010) *The ACSM Guidelines for Exercising Testing and Prescription 8th Edition*, Lippincott, Williams and Wilkins, Philadelphia, PA

Anderson, O. (2004) Peak Performance Special Training Report

Baechle, T.R. and Earle, R. (Eds) (2000) *Essentials of Strength Training and Conditioning 2nd Edition*, Human Kinetics, Champaign, IL

Brock, D.W. et al. (2010) 'Exercise training prevents regain of visceral fat for 1 year following weight loss' *Obesity (Silver Spring),* 18(4), 690-5

Brooks, D.S. (1998) *Program Design for Personal Trainers: Bridging Theory into Application,* Human Kinetics, Champaign, IL

Boutcher, S. (2011) 'High-Intensity Intermittent Exercise and Fat Loss', *Journal of Obesity*. Doi: 10.1155/2011/868305

Clark M.A. and Corn R.J. (2001) *Optimum Performance Training for the Fitness Professional,* National Academy of Sports Medicine, Thousand Oaks, CA

Donnelly, J.E. et al. (2009) 'Appropriate Physical Activity Intervention Strategies for Weight Loss and Prevention of Weight Regain for Adults', *Medicine and Science in Sports and Exercise*, 41(2), 459-71

Heyward, V.H. (2006) *Advanced Fitness Assessment and Exercise Prescription 5th Edition*, Human Kinetics, Champaign, IL

Irving, B.A. et al. (2008) 'Effect of exercise training intensity on abdominal visceral fat and body composition', *Medicine and Science in Sports and Exercise,* 40(11), 1863-72.

King et al. (2001) 'A comparison of high intensity vs. low intensity exercise on body composition in overweight women'. *Medicine and Science in Sports and Exercise*, 33, A2421

McArdle, W.D., Katch, F.I. And Katch, V.L. (2010) *Exercise Physiology: Energy, Nutrition and Human Performance 7th Edition,* Lippincott Williams and Wilkins, Philadelphia, PA

Saris, W.H.N. et al. (2003) 'How much physical activity is enough to prevent unhealthy weight gain? Outcome of the IASO 1st Stock Conference and consensus statement', *Obesity Review,* 4(2), 101-14

Schuenke, M.D., Mikat, R.P. and McBride, J.M. (2002) 'Effect of an acute period of resistance exercise on excess post-exercise oxygen consumption: implications for body mass management', *European Journal of Applied Physiology,* 86(5), 411-7

Sleamaker, R. and Browning, R. (1996) *SERIOUS Training for Endurance Athletes 2nd Edition*, Human Kinetics, Champaign, IL

Trapp, E.G., Chisholm, D.J., Freund, J. and Boutcher, S.H. (2008) 'The effects of high-intensity intermittent exercise training on fat loss and fasting insulin levels of young women', *International Journal of Obesity,* 32(4), 684-91

Tremblay et al. (1994) 'Impact of exercise intensity on body fatness and skeletal muscle metabolism', *Metabolism,* 43: 814-18

Wallace, J.P. and Ray, S. (2009) 'Obesity' in Durstine et al. (Eds.) *ACSM's Exercise Management for Persons with Chronic Diseases and Disabilities 3rd Edition*, Human Kinetics, Champaign, IL

Whyte, L.J., Gill, J.M.R. and Cathcart, A.J. (2010) 'Effect of 2 weeks of sprint interval training on health-related outcomes in sedentary overweight/obese men', *Metabolism Clinical and Experimental*, 59(10), 1421-28

Wescott, W.L. (2003) *Senior Strength* Fitpro Feb/March

Wilmore, J.H. and Costill, D.L. (2004) *Physiology of Sport and Exercise 3rd Edition*, Human Kinetics, Champaign, IL

Wilmore, J.H., Costill, D.L. and Kennedy W.L. (2008) *Physiology of Sport and Exercise 4th Edition* Human Kinetics, Champaign, IL

THE CENTRAL YMCA GUIDES SERIES

Happy and Healthy: A collection of trustworthy advice on health, fitness and wellbeing topics

UK
http://www.centralymcaguides.com/hhct2

US
http://www.centralymcaguides.com/hhct

The Scientific Approach to Exercise for Fat Loss: How to get in shape and shed unwanted fat by using healthy and scientifically proven techniques

UK
http://www.centralymcaguides.com/sael2

US
http://www.centralymcaguides.com/sael

The Need to Know Guide to Nutrition for Exercise: How your food and drink can help you to achieve your workout goals

UK
http://www.centralymcaguides.com/ngne2

US
http://www.centralymcaguides.com/ngne

***The Need to Know Guide to Nutrition and Healthy Eating:** The perfect starter to eating well or how to eat the right foods, stay in shape and stick to a healthy diet*

UK http://www.centralymcaguides.com/gnhe2

US http://www.centralymcaguides.com/gnhe

***Tri Harder - The A to Z of Triathlon for Improvers:** The triathlon competitors' guide to training and improving your running, cycling and swimming times*

UK http://www.centralymcaguides.com/thtc2

US http://www.centralymcaguides.com/thtc

***20 Full Body Training Programmes for Exercise Lovers:** An essential guide to boosting your general fitness, strength, power and endurance*

UK http://www.centralymcaguides.com/tpel2

US http://www.centralymcaguides.com/tpel

***Run, Jump, Climb, Crawl:** The essential training guide for obstacle racing enthusiasts, or how to get fit, stay safe and prepare for the toughest mud runs on the planet*

UK http://www.centralymcaguides.com/rjc2

US http://www.centralymcaguides.com/rjc

Gardening for Health: The Need to Know Guide to the Health Benefits of Horticulture

UK
http://www.centralymcaguides.com/gfhh2

US
http://www.centralymcaguides.com/gfhh

New Baby, New You: The Need to Know Guide to Postnatal Health and Happiness - How to return to exercise and get back in shape after giving birth

UK
http://www.centralymcaguides.com/nbny2

US
http://www.centralymcaguides.com/nbny

The Need to Know Guide to Life with a Toddler and a Newborn: How to prepare for and cope with the day to day challenge of raising two young children

UK
http://www.centralymcaguides.com/ngtn2

US
http://www.centralymcaguides.com/ngtn

50 Games for Active Toddlers: Quick everyday hints and tips to keep toddlers active, healthy and occupied

UK
http://www.centralymcaguides.com/50uk

US
http://www.centralymcaguides.com/50us

Exercise and Nutrition 3 Book Bundle

UK
http://www.centralymcaguides.com/enb2

US
http://www.centralymcaguides.com/enb

Obstacle Racing Preparation 3 Book Bundle

UK
http://www.centralymcaguides.com/orpb2

US
http://www.centralymcaguides.com/orpb

Nutrition and Fat Loss 3 Book Bundle

UK
http://www.centralymcaguides.com/nflb2

US
http://www.centralymcaguides.com/nflb

Mums' Health 3 Book Bundle

UK
http://www.centralymcaguides.com/mhb2

US
http://www.centralymcaguides.com/mhb

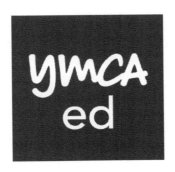

Discover more books and ebooks of interest to you and find out about the range of work we do at the forefront of health, fitness and wellbeing.

www.centralymcaguides.com

Printed in Great Britain
by Amazon